New Gout Relief Diet

I0429076

"Discover New Gout Remedies for Eliminating Uric and Body Acids"

Individual with gout

Microscopic view of joint fluid

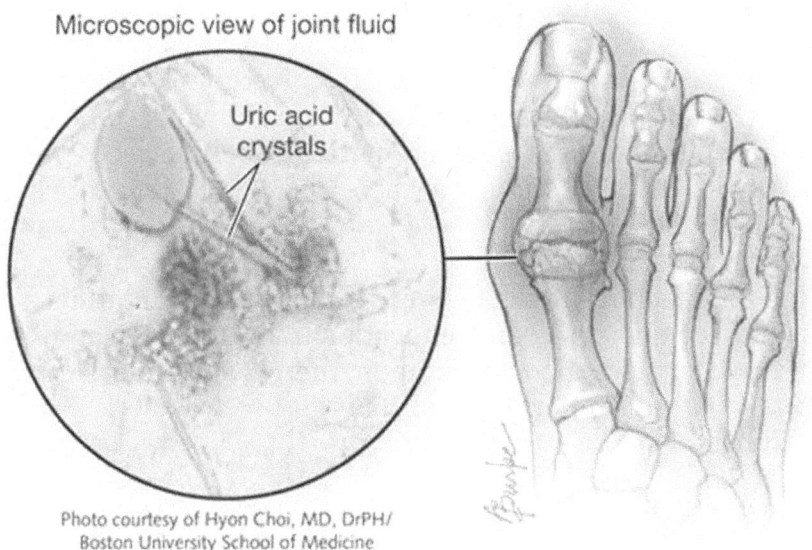

Uric acid crystals

Photo courtesy of Hyon Choi, MD, DrPH/
Boston University School of Medicine

By Kevin Reed, Nutritional Consultant

New Gout Relief Diet © 2014, by Kevin Reed

ISBN-13: 978-1500555191

ISBN-10: 1500555193

Disclaimer and Terms of Use: The Author and Publisher has strived to be as accurate and complete as possible in the creation of this book, notwithstanding the fact that he does not warrant or represent at any time that the contents within are accurate due to the rapidly changing nature of the Internet. While all attempts have been made to verify information provided in this publication, the Author and Publisher assumes no responsibility for errors, omissions, or contrary interpretation of the subject matter herein. Any perceived slights of specific persons, peoples, or organizations are unintentional.

This book is not intended as medical advice or treatment and should be considered only educational information, and if you feel like you need a doctor opinion, then you should seek it. Printed in the United States of America

Table Of Contents

1: Discover Why You Have Gout

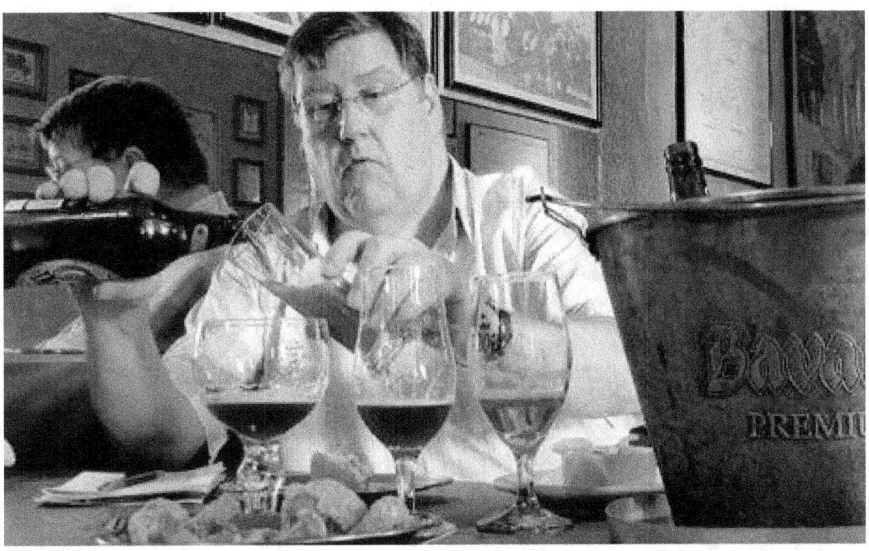

It was thought at one time that gout was a disease that only the elderly, rich, and others who over ate developed this condition. However, with the increase in processed food and the appearance of junk food, those that favored this food became victims of an acid body and of excess uric acid.

The real cause of gout is an imbalance of the acid-alkaline balance in your body. There are two different types of acids that you need to be concerned with and eliminate when you have gout – uric acid and acid body.

How this uric acid and an acid-alkaline imbalance occurs, how it creates gout, and what you can do about it is what this book is all about.

Once you rebalance your acids, you not only get rid of gout, but you create an alkaline body that is less susceptible to disease.

Gout and Arthritis

Gout is expressed as form of arthritis, "gouty arthritis," muscle or tissue pain in your body, but is not arthritis. I'm sure many of you have had some form of pain in your legs or calves that woke you up, at night giving you agonizing pain, if you move your legs. Now, this might not be gout, but this is the type of pain that gout sufferers experience, but only more painful and mostly located in their joints.

If you have gout, you may experience piercing sharp pain in your joints, toes, ankles, knees, shoulders or elbows. This pain comes from the formation of needle-like uric crystals that precipitate and attach themselves to your cartilage, muscle tissue, skin tissue or synovial pouches in your joints.

These uric crystals come from excess uric acid that travels throughout your blood, and which drops out of your blood to form crystals. Not all people with excess uric acid develop gout. But, if they do, there are other illnesses that they may develop, without knowing it.

Uric acid is not only responsible for gout, but is the seed for kidney stones.

Here are some conditions that make you more susceptible to gout.

Family History

First of all, studies have shown that if your family members suffer from gout, your chance of having gout are 20% higher. The reason for this might come from the way you developed your eating habit, as a child. Most family members all eat the same food and may develop unhealthy eating habits.

Your Medical conditions

There are various medical conditions that can increase your risk of developing gout. When you have an illness and or are taking drugs, this situation means that you have an acid body. When you have an acid body, you are more prone to having gout. Here are four conditions that contribute to gout.

High blood pressure (hypertension)
Diabetes, both type 1 diabetes and type 2 diabetes
Kidney disease
Hypothyroidism
Having high levels of fat and cholesterol levels in your blood
Obesity
Some cancers
Other illnesses

See a Doctor

There are many other body conditions or illnesses that may appear as gout. So, see your doctor, to confirm it is gout and not some other serious condition.

2: Get Real Information On Gout

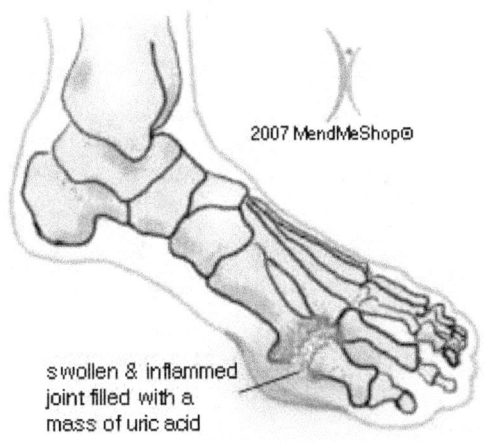

2007 MendMeShop®

swollen & inflammed
joint filled with a
mass of uric acid

Gout is considered an inflammatory disease. When inflammation occurs anywhere in your body, it occurs because something is irritating, burning, or damaging your body's tissues.

Gout is an inflammation of various bone joints and is considered a form of arthritis. This inflammation occurs when **monosodium urate monohydrate crystals** deposit or precipitate in your joints or in the joint synovial fluid. When these crystals form, they contain sharp points, which tear or cut into cartilage, bone ligaments, and tissue, causing great pain and discomfort.

These crystals can also deposit in major organs, causing major damage. For this reason, it's important to take action on this disease to eliminate it and stop its return.

This gout pain often comes at night, when you are deep asleep. The sharp pains appear in your toes, joints or calves. Any movement of your legs increases the pain. The pain can be unbearable at times.

Gout pain may last for days or even weeks, and the time between attacks can be weeks or years.

Purine is Uric Acid

Gout also occurs when an excess of meat or other food, which contain a high level of purines is eaten.

So, what are purines? Purines occur in all foods and plants. They help to form the chemical structure of genes. When you eat food, the genes in this food are broken down, during digestion and purine is released. This purine is now uric acid. It remains in the blood, dissolved and harmless.

When your old cells die and decomposed, purine is released into your blood. This is another source of uric acid.

Typically, 70% of the urate produced daily is eliminated by your kidneys in urine. The other 30% is routed to your liver and moved into your gallbladder and into your colon, where it is removed by your stools.

When too much purine food is eaten and uric acid is produced, hyperuricaemia, by your body, your body has to figure out how to get rid of it.

Too much uric acid can also remain in your body, if your kidneys are not functioning properly. Your kidneys will not remove the 70%. If your liver doesn't remove the 30% it is required to, excess uric acid can remain in your blood.

What Causes Urate Crystals to Form?

Urate crystals form when you have too much uric acid in your blood, but not all people with an excess of uric acid form urate crystals.

Urate crystals form when you have an imbalance in your acid-alkaline levels. When you have an excess of acid in your body, uric acid will tend to precipitate and form crystals.

So, if you have an alkaline body, your chances of having gout are considerably less. If you have an acid body, your chances of having gout are higher.

Gout Attacks

Gout attacks occur for a short time, but are quite painful, when they occur. In some cases, a gout attack can happen on occasion or frequently. When gout attacks occur frequently or take some time to disappear, these attacks can cause weakening, deformation, or destruction of your joints.

How Does Uric Acid Buildup In Your Blood?

In normal people, the amount of uric acid that is created from daily eating, body exercise, or cell activities is expelled from the body, and no gout is ever experienced. However, in some people,

1. Their kidneys do not eliminate enough uric acid and the uric blood level rises.

2. They over exercise causing an excess of uric acid to build-up in their blood.

3. They become dehydrated, by not drinking plenty of water, during the day or during strenuous exercise. Less liquid in your body cause uric acid to rise. More frequent urination reduces the uric acid in your blood.

4. They become ill or come down with more infections than normal, causing more uric acid in their blood

5. They have hypothyroidism, leukemia, psoriasis, or lymphoma.

6. They injured a joint creating a weak point where uric acid crystals can deposit easily.

7. They start to lose weight too fast, using various diet programs, which interrupt the excretion of uric acid through their urine.

8. Their overweight condition leads to an increase chance of a gout attack. Extra pounds cause the body to produce more uric acid and also to block the excretion of this uric acid from the body.

9. They have excess stress or are extra nervous, which cause uric acid to rise in the blood.

10. They drink up to a dozen cans of beer or 2 ½ liters. Alcohol slows down the excretion of uric acid in the kidneys.

11. They drink an excess of sodas, which contain sugar or fructose and this causes uric acid.

12. They have a previous joint injury.

13. They use recreational drugs or medical drugs for other diseases.

14. They have a tumor.

15. They have lead poisoning.

16. They have a digestive enzyme deficiency causing poor digestion and excess acid waste in the stomach.

Gout is not always just a symptom that comes for a short time. Many people experience gout for weeks and sometimes for

extended periods.

Some Medical Treatments for Gout

If you wish to use medical treatment for your gout, here is what you can expect.

The recommended treatment for a gout attack is the use NSAIDs or Non-steroidal Anti-inflammatory Drugs, such as naproxen, 500mg for every 10 hours.

Nonsteroidal Anti-Inflammatories (NSAIDs) - Indocin, Indomethicin, Ibuprofen, Naproxen, Naprosyn, Aleve – These drugs decrease gout inflammation and pain. Their side effects are nausea, abdominal pain or bleeding, indigestion, dizziness, and stomach ulcers.

If you can't tolerate NSAIDs, then corticosteroids are recommended. If you don't like corticosteroids, then colchicine is the drug to take. Your doctor will help you with the drug you need.

3: Foods That Create Uric Acid

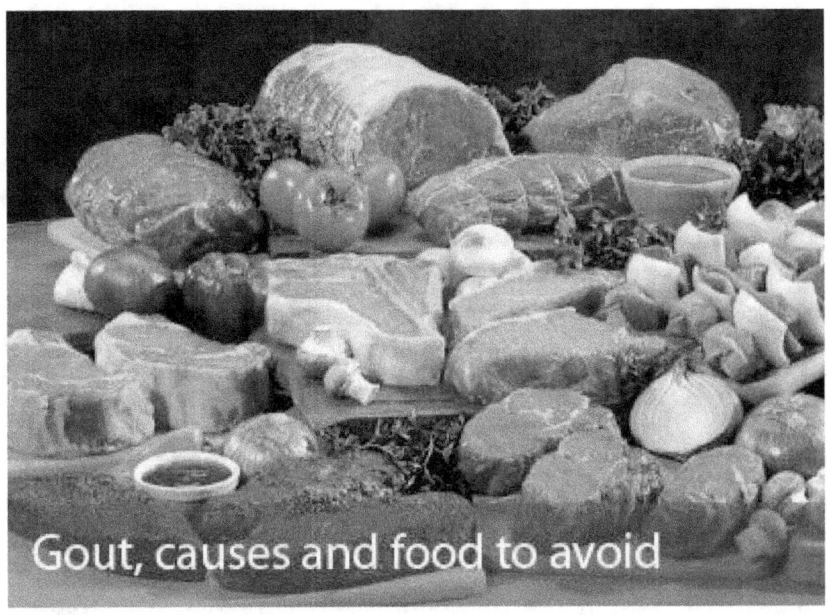

Gout, causes and food to avoid

Here is what you can expect from a diet. The food you eat must minimize the creation of uric acid and acid body.

Uric Acid

Fats or fatty foods play an important part in gout. If you have a diet high in fats, these fats prevent your kidneys from removing the amount of uric acid that it should. The result is that an excess of uric acid remains in your blood.

In this chapter are the foods that are high in purine, and that you should cut back on, if you are prone to gout attacks. You don't have to eliminate these foods from your diet forever. In fact, you may just need to limit the amount that you eat.

Meat

All animal meat contains purine, such as red meat, organ meat, meat extracts, and some fish. So cut back on these meats.

Some of the fish to avoid are herring, sardines, and mussels.

Alcohol

Beer has always been suggested to avoid, when you have gout. However, it is also best to eliminate all alcohol beverages, when you are in a gout attack.

Baked Goods

Baked goods, which have yeast, also contain purines and should be avoided.

Soft Drinks

Soft drinks and other sugary drinks, which are high in fructose, can cause an excess of uric acid in your blood. Just one or two drinks a day can cause you uric acid problems. Fruit juices can also cause uric problems, if they are not fresh and don't have enough fiber in them.

Foods to avoid, if you have gout

Here is a list of food that you need to minimize or eliminate from your diet.

- Avoid or minimize the use Scallops, herring, tuna, anchovies and meat during a gout attack.

- Reduce the use of red meat, chicken, pork, turkey or lamb

- Avoid eating animal skin and fatty meat.

- Limit the use of bouillon, commercially prepared gravies or soups.

- Limit your use of chocolates

- Avoid sodas and sugar, corn syrup, or fructose sweetened drinks.

- Avoid sweetbreads, chips, sugary products, and junk food

- Avoid or minimize the use asparagus, cauliflower, spinach, and mushrooms, peas, beans and legumes.

- Eliminate completely liver and kidney meat

- Stop drinking Beer tea, coffee, cocoa

- Minimize your use of oats, but you can use them occasionally

4: The Gout Diet to Reduce Pain

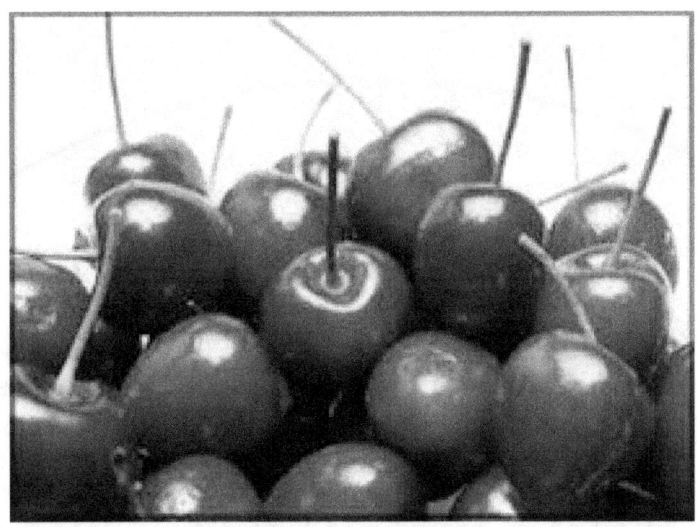

There are many foods that you can eat to help you clear your gout. For gout pain that occurs for 15 to 30 minutes a day or more, apply the principles listed in the chapters on burning acid. These practices will eliminate and cure your infrequent gout attacks. In addition, these practices are the foundation of creating a healthy body.

If you have gout attacks that remain for days, then you need to follow the food practices, in the previous chapter, that will not aggravate your gout.

Increase your consumption of vegetables and fruits in all forms. When you do this, you are helping your body excrete purine chemicals from your body and create an alkaline body. Your basic diet should be a moderate protein and fat intake, with no internal organs.

Dairy products are good to eat such as,

- Milk and non-fermented milk products
- Eggs whites, hard boiled for the egg whites
- Cottage cheese, mozzarella cheese
- Whey protein
- Shrimp, lobster, eel, and crab in moderation.
- Complex carbohydrates, brown rice, wheat bread, pasta
- Citrus fruits, non-sweeten juices
- Herbal teas, Coffee
- Water

Egg whites, milk, and whey protein do not have purines, and this is why they are on the list of foods to eat. However, yogurt and aged cheeses are not on the eat list.

Eating low-fat dairy is recommended for gout. Use skim milk or low-fat yogurt.

Water

Drinking plenty of water is necessary, to clear your gout. This increases the frequency of urination, and when you urinate, your kidneys excrete uric acid from your blood.

Purines in Food

Purines cannot be entirely avoided, because they occur in produce and other foods. In addition, they are created in your body as a result of recycling dead cells.

Apple

Eat at least two apples per day to neutralize uric acid. Eat them between meals and not after a meal. Apples will also give you relief from gout pain and reduce its inflammation.

Apple and Carrots

Eating carrots and apples is a great way to reduce gout acid and pain. One way to get daily relief is to juice apples and carrots together. Make a mixture of 1:1, or make 3/4 apple juice with 1/4 carrot juice.

Use carrots in any way that you can, either raw or cooked. The more carrots you eat the fewer issues you will have with gout.

Avocados

Avocados are high in essential fatty acids that help to reduce body pain.

Celery

It is recommended that you take a supplement of celery seeds, when you have gout. While waiting to get the seeds, you can eat 4-5 celery sticks per day with the leaves. This will help you to lower your uric blood levels.

Juice of Cucumber, Carrot, Spinach

A juicer is a great tool to have. You can create all kinds of juices, when you have to. Creating a juice of cucumber, carrots and spinach can help you get rid of a lot of uric acid. Cucumber is a strong diuretic and will help to produce more urine.

Add some apple to this cucumber mixture, to sweeten up this juice. Then, you will be able to drink more of it.

Artichoke

When you eat artichokes, they have the ability to reduce the production of uric acid, in your body. Not all people like artichokes and you have to develop a taste for them.

Artichokes have excellent health benefits, such as body detoxifying, cholesterol lowering, and liver repair.

Bananas

Bananas can treat gout. They are high in potassium and other minerals, which convert uric crystals into liquid. Eat only two to three bananas per day. Choose those bananas that are not over ripe, but just right for eating.

Red or Black Cherries or Strawberries

Tart Cherries contain anti-inflammatory and potent antioxidants chemicals, such as flavonols and the Anthocyanins, which is an anti-inflammatory antioxidant.

This is a well-known remedy for gout, but researchers have found it hard to discover why cherries relieve gout. Despite many stories about how people were helped with gout by drinking or eating cherries, there are still some people that are not helped. If cherries don't reduce your gout symptoms, then move on to eating other foods that do.

In a well-documented story, 1950, Ludwig Blau, Ph.D. reported in the *Texas Reports on Biology and Medicine* that he cured his gout that had him in a wheel chair. He did this by eating or drinking cherries every day. He found that as long as he ate cherries, he had no gout pain. He used 6–8 cherries per day.

More cherries can be eaten, but 6 to 8 are the minimum. You can also use cherry extract, to prepare a cherry drink or to add to a fruit smoothie.

Fresh cherries always work best for gout, since the nutrients are in higher concentration. But, frozen ones also work.

Pineapples and Juice

Eat pineapples and pineapple juice to ease your joint pain. Pineapples, with the protein digestive enzyme bromelain, help to reduce joint inflammation.

Grapes

Grapes are high in minerals that move your body toward alkalinity. Any slight movement towards an alkaline body means fewer uric acid will form uric crystals.

This little fruit will reduce the acidity of uric acid and then helps to eliminate it through your kidneys.

Nuts

Eat a variety of nuts, but do it in moderation.

Fish

You need to eat some type of fish. It has been found that fish oil provides lubricant to your joints. Without some form of lubricant, your joints will wear down your cartilage as they rub together. You can supplement with a good fish oil capsule, to provide this lubricant.

Seaweed

All seaweed is beneficial in curing gout. These foods contain a high level of minerals. The balance of these minerals is in a way that your body needs them. They will make your body more alkaline, because of the calcium, potassium, and sodium they contain.

Vegetables and Fruits

Concentrate on vegetables, like sweet potatoes, squashes, cabbage, and potatoes. You can prepare them any way you like. Also, eat many of the other vegetables you like.

Both vegetables and fruits are high in antioxidants and minerals. Antioxidants help fight off damage to your joints and reduce inflammation. Minerals make your body less acidic and keep uric acid in solution and not in crystal form.

Vegetable Juices

If you have a juicer, then you are prepared to fight various diseases. By creating the juice of a combination of vegetables, you can produce a high alkaline drink that will keep your gout away.

Dandelion Leaves - Vegetable Salads

When you make a green salad, add some dandelion, kale, and spinach leaves. All the salad leaves are high in minerals and help make your body more alkaline.

5: Natural Remedies You Should Use for Gout

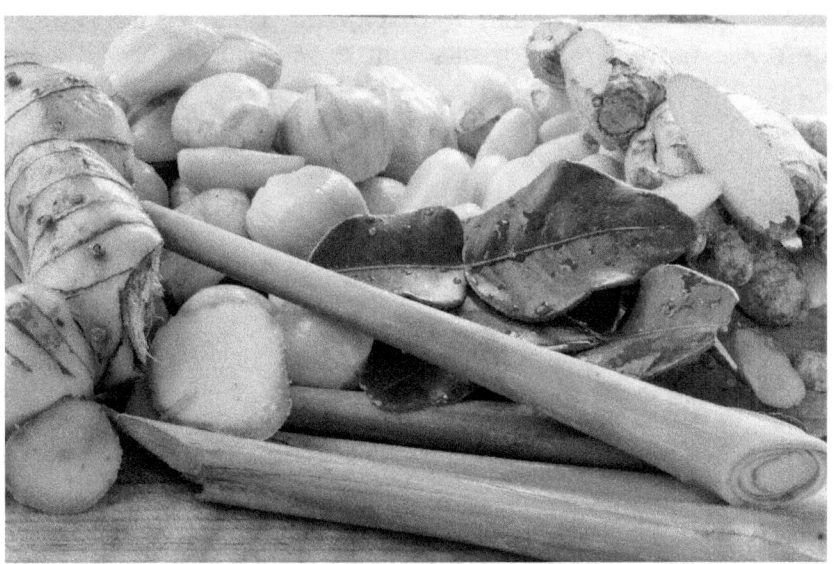

Creating Uric Acid

Losing weight leads to substances the stop the excretion of your uric acid. Keeping your weight or losing it at a slower rate can help reduce gout attacks. Don't eat less the 1700 1900 calories per day, but this just a guide line.

It has been found that one of the best approaches for eliminating gout or for controlling it is to move your body from an acid state to an alkaline state. This is done by concentrating on foods that produce an alkaline residue, when your cells metabolize nutrients. You can increase your transition from acid to alkaline, by taking alkaline minerals with your meals.

Here some of the most effective natural remedies that have been used to minimize or eliminate gout pain.

Alfalfa

Alfalfa is packed with minerals, which will make your body more alkaline. This is one of the things that will help you cure your gout. You can take it in capsule form or in powder. There are many green drinks that contain alfalfa, and many other greens that make an excellent morning drink for your gout.

Apple Cider Vinegar

Apple cider vinegar has been found to work for many ailments. For gout, here's what you need to do.

Take 2 teaspoons of organic apple cider vinegar and add 2 teaspoons of honey. Do these two times a day. This remedy will reduce your gout pain, within a few hours.

You can mix 1 to 2 tablespoon of apple cider vinegar in 8 oz. of water and drink it, once per day. You can add a bit of honey, if you need to.

Baking Soda

Baking soda helps to lower the amount of uric acid in your blood. When you do this, you will get relief from joint pain. Here's how to use it.

Place 1/2 teaspoon of baking soda in 8 oz of water and drink it. You can do this three times a day only. If you have high blood pressure, **don't use this remedy.**

Limit your use of this remedy, since it will change the pH of your stomach acid.

Celery Seed

Here is another remedy that is great for gout pain. You can eat

one tablespoon of celery seeds per day, or you can take celery seed capsules. Celery seeds have the compound "Sedanolide," which is used in other herbal remedies for gout inflammation.

Dandelion Extract

Dandelion extract is useful for gout, since it contains a lot of **Potassium**. This mineral can neutralize body acids and reduce your body acid load, making your body more alkaline. When this happens, uric acid is more likely to remain in solution, instead of precipitating into damaging crystal deposits.

If you can't get dandelion extract, try getting the herb and making a tea. Allow the herb to sit in hot water for 10 to 15 minutes to make it stronger. Add some honey to give it more flavor.

Devil's Claw

Devil's claw will provide you anti-inflammatory benefits and lower uric acid levels, which can help with your gout pain.
If you have diabetes or are taking a blood-thinning drug **do not take this herb**.

Boswellia

Boswellia is an Indian herb that has shown to control arthritis. It reduces inflammation and promotes circulation in the affected areas. It is good for gout inflammation.

Drinking Water

Drinking a lot of water, when you have gout is a smart idea. Uric acid is removed by your kidneys through your urine. The more you urinate the less uric acid you have in your body. The more uric acid you have in your body the more likely you will form uric acid crystals in your joints.

So, drink 6 – 7 glasses of water per day. If you eat fruits and fruit juices without sugar or fructose, you can count this as water. Herbal teas can, also, be counted as water, but not regular tea.

Ice Water

Using an ice pack on your gout inflammation can quickly reduce your pain. Use this idea with other remedies listed here. An ice pack will only provide temporary relief.

You can also make an ice bath, which is not fully loaded with ice, but just enough to create a cold bath that will remove some of the pain and burning joint sensation. Use this bath until it starts to reach room temperature.

Epsom Salt

A warm foot bath with Epsom salt is another good gout remedy. In a foot tub, add warm water and 1/2 cup of Epsom salt. If you need more salt, add a slight more. Soak your foot or feet, until the water gets cold. Do this once a week. You will be absorbing many of the minerals in the Epsom salt, which will make your body more alkaline.

Garlic

Garlic should be used in all cooking and taken in supplements, because of its long list of health benefits it provides. For gout, it has been shown to reduce joint pain and gout symptoms.

Ginger Root

Ginger root has anti-inflammatory properties. Here's how to use it.

1. Drink a glass of ginger root tea every day.

2. Use ginger root in your cooking every day.

3. Create a paste of ginger root and apply it to the affected area.

4. Ground 1/3 cup of ginger and place it in a foot tub of warm water. Soak your affected foot for 30 minutes. This will help to eliminate some of your uric acid. Rinse your foot off with water, after your 30 minutes.

Green Powder or Capsules

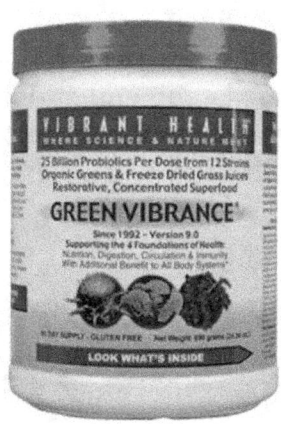

A good green called **Green Vibrance** provides you with a variety of green grasses. It's these grasses that contain the minerals and other nutrients that you need to eliminate gout.

Green Vibrance contains organic barley, oat, wheat, Kamut, alfalfa sprouts, broccoli sprouts, spirulina, chlorella, rice bran, and many more vegetables.

Grape seed or pine bark extracts.

These extracts are high in antioxidants and will neutralize damaging free radicals, in your joints and tissue. They work as an anti-inflammatory remedy. You can put this extract over the affected joint.

Juniper Oil

Place a compress of juniper oil on your affected area. Juniper oil will help to break down the uric crystals.

Placing this on the affected area will help break down the toxic deposits.

Lemon Juice

Lemon juice is a powerful remedy for gout. Even though its juice is acidic, when this juice is metabolized at the cell level, it creates what is called an alkaline ash or residue, which will neutralize acid. This makes your body more alkaline, and your uric acid tends to remains as liquid, when your body is more alkaline.

First, when you first wake up, drink 8 oz. of distilled water with the juice of one lemon and do this three times per day. Add a little honey to sweeten this drink, if you like.

Here's another way to use lemon. Juice one lemon and add it to 1/2 teaspoon of baking soda. Mix these ingredients, and then add it to 8 oz. of water. Afterwards, drink up.

Milk Thistle

Milk Thistle is known as a liver tonic and can protect the liver from toxins, as found in gout medications. You need a healthy liver, so it can move uric acid out through your gallbladder and colon.

Ruby Reds

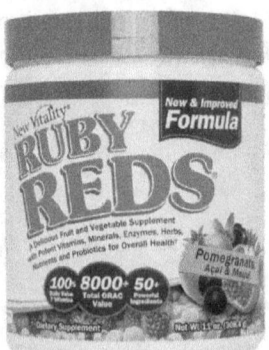

Ruby Reds is a powder supplement that contains over 50 natural ingredients of fruits, vegetables, fiber, probiotics and digestive enzymes. This is an excellent powder that you can add to your smoothies or to create a morning drink with juice. This supplement gives you an excellent source of antioxidants and minerals that
will help you with your gout.

This is a Delicious Fruit and Vegetable Supplement with the right vitamins, minerals, enzymes, herbs, nutrients and probiotics for overall health. One glass gives you the antioxidant power of 13 servings of fruits and vegetables.

Rutin

Rutin is good for reducing gout inflammation. It also reduces uric acid and prevents it from forming joint crystals.

You can buy rutin as a supplement, which is a nice way to get it.

Willow Bark

Willow contains compounds as salicylates from which aspirin is created. Using a strong tea of willow can help you relieve pain and inflammation.

Yucca Herb Stock Leaf

Yucca Herb has antioxidants, anti inflammatory, free-radical scavenging, anti-arthritic properties, and anti-inflammatory benefits. Drink this every day, for gout.

Turmeric Root

Turmeric has benefits for arthritis because of its anti-inflammatory properties and thus helps reduce gout pain. It does this by the curcumin that it has, which blocks prostaglandins that produce pain in your body. This chemical process is similar to the action of aspirin and ibuprofen, but not as strong.

You can take turmeric root in capsules to get a high dose. Or you add a curry dish to your weekly diet.

6: Supplements to Help Cure Gout

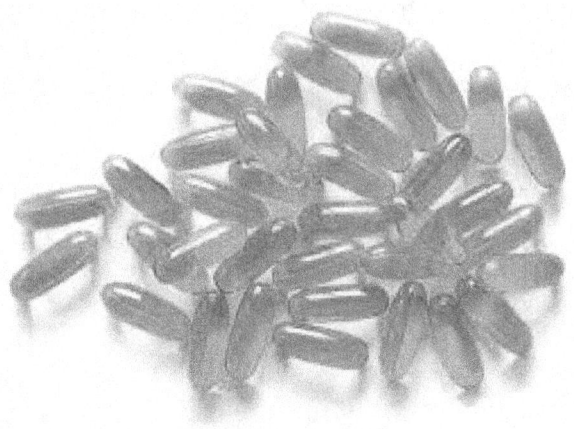

There is one supplement that you need to avoid, niacin. This supplement can create a gout attack, since the nicotinic acid created in your blood competes with uric acid in your kidneys to be excreted. If you are using niacin under a doctor's care for cardiovascular conditions, check with your doctor about eliminating it, if you have gout.

There are not very many supplements to take for gout. But, of the few that are, vitamin C is one that you should be taking. Vitamin C is used by your body for a variety of different body conditions, so you should be taking it, even though you may not have gout.

Vitamin C supplements

In a 2009 vitamin C study, vitamin C showed a reduced risk of developing gout. This study had 46,994 men who were followed for several years. It compared men with a vitamin C intake of less than 250 mg a day. The result was that those men whose vitamin C intake of 1,000-1,499 mg per day had a 34% lower risk of gout.

And, for those men who took 1,500+ mg per day, they had a 45% lower risk of gout.

Taking vitamin C for gout makes a lot sense. It appears that vitamin C works by reducing the uric acid in your blood. It may do this by excreting more of it out your urine than normal.

Folic Acid

Folic acid is used in your body in the breakdown of proteins. It also blocks the action of an enzyme that is responsible for forming uric acid.

You should use from 200 to 400 micrograms per day.

No side effects have been reported, when taking high doses of folic acid. Folic acid in these high doses has been shown to be as effective as the drug allopurinol.

High doses of folic acid should be taken with a doctor's care, since they can mask the deficiency of vitamin B12.

Alpha Lipoic Acid

There are chemicals called leukotrienes, which are involved in joint inflammation. You can reduce this inflammation by taking alpha lipoic acid with vitamin E and selenium. Here's the dose to take:

Alpha lipoic Acid, 50 to 800 mg per day
Vitamin E, 200 to 400 IU per day
Selenium, 200 micrograms per day

Bromelain

Bromelain is a digestive enzyme found in pineapple and is an effective anti-inflammatory.

Take Bromelain, 500 to 1,500 GDUs (Gelatin digestion units)

Essential fatty Acids

The essential fatty acids, omega-3, omega-6, and omega-9 are anti-inflammatory substances. You can get them in a variety of sources, such as fish oil, flax seed oil, evening primrose, olive oil, and other oils. It is best to use fish oil for gout.
Use Fish oil, 1,200 to 2,000 mg per day

7: How Minerals Burn Acid and Relieve Gout

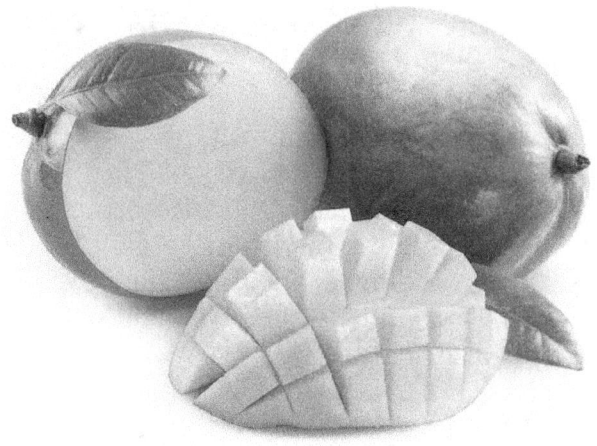

Minerals

Moving your body more toward alkalinity is what will give you the best health. When you have gout problems, getting more minerals in your body is the first step. An alkaline body prevents your body from becoming ill and forming deadly diseases, like joint problems, organ degradation, body pain, skin eruptions, cancer, and system weaknesses. If you are already sick, then all the chemicals inside fruits and vegetables will help revive you to better health. This is provided that your tissue damage has not gone beyond repair.

Uric acid also has higher solubility in solutions of alkali hydroxides and their carbonates than in acidic media. So making your body more alkaline, is what you need to do to reduce or eliminate gout.

The minerals most important in changing and maintaining your body in an alkaline condition are sodium, potassium, solutions. Other minerals such as chloride, calcium, phosphorus, magnesium, and sulfur are also critical in making your body alkaline.

Acid Binding

Acid Binding Fruits With Alkaline Minerals

In the list below are fruits and vegetables with alkaline minerals that create acid binding salts in your body, used to neutralize acid wastes. Foods above 50% in value are more acid binding, which means they will more trap or bind with acid wastes. Foods below 50% are more acid producing and are called alkaline binding, since they tie up or bind with alkaline minerals. This means a loss of alkaline minerals that you need to neutralize acids.

To create an alkaline body, you need to eat 80% acid binding food and 20% alkaline binding food. Work towards this end and you will slowly move your body from acid to alkaline.
Here is the list of foods to eat in the order of priority. Acid binding means that these fruits will bind and eliminate your body acids.

Fruits

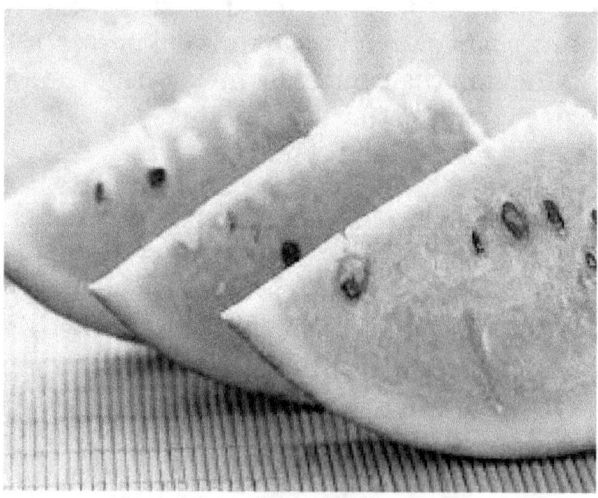

Fruits at 100% Acid Binding – Best Fruits To Eat
Lemons, melons – any type, watermelon

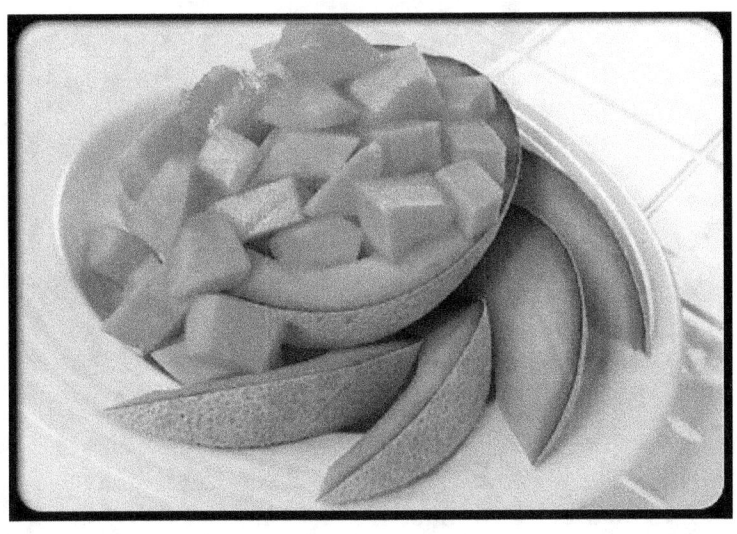

Fruits at 93% Acid Binding – Great Fruits To Eat
Cantaloupes, dried dates, dried figs, limes, mango, papaya

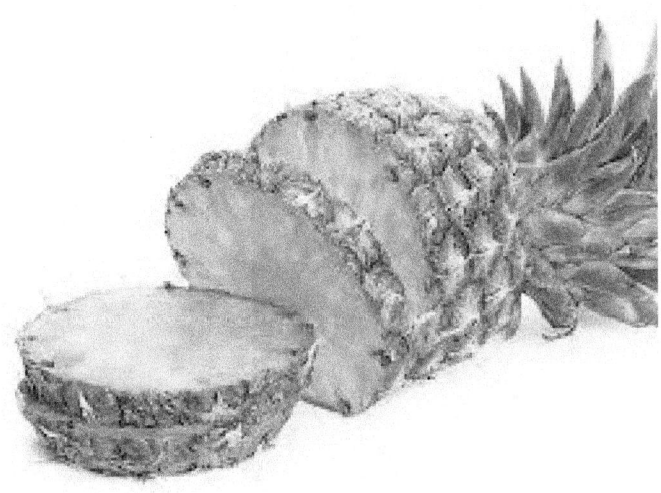

Fruits at 87% Acid Binding – Still Great Fruits To Eat
Kiwis, passion Fruit, pineapples, raisins, umeboshi plums

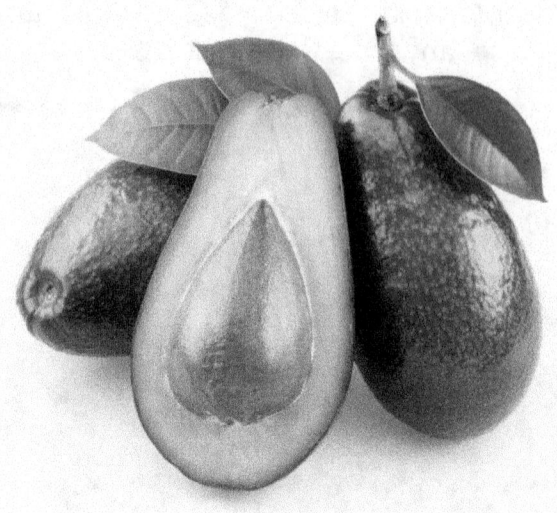

Fruits at 80% Acid Binding – Eat These Fruits
Apricots, avocados, bananas, fresh dates, fresh figs, currants, gooseberries grapes, guavas, kumquats, nectarines, pears, persimmons, quince, berries, cactus

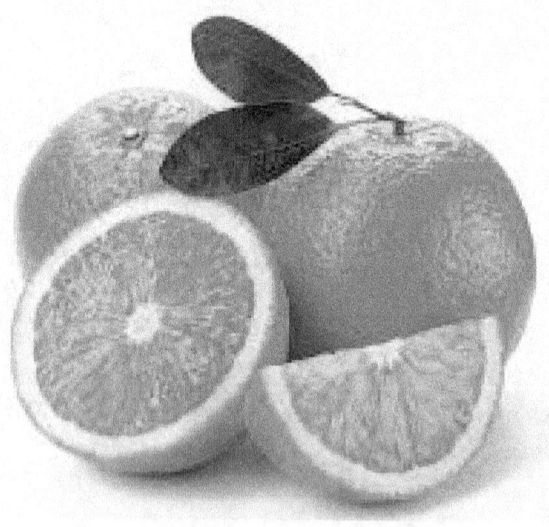

Fruits 73% Acid Binding – Still Fruits To Eat
Apples, oranges, peaches, pomegranate, raspberries, sour grapes, strawberries, carob

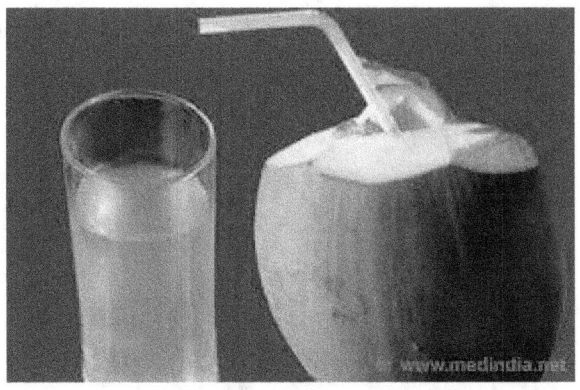

Fruits at 67% Acid Binding – Still Neutralizes Acids
Cherries, fresh coconut

Herbal Teas From Leaves at 73% to 86% acid binding
Alfalfa, mint, sage, spearmint, raspberry, strawberry comfrey
All Herbs and Spices at 67% to 73% Acid Binding

Fruits 40% to 47% - Eat less of these fruits
Blueberries, cranberries, plums, prunes

All Juices from a juicer 100% Acid Binding

Vegetables

Here is the list of vegetables to eat for gout in order of priority.
All of these vegetables will neutralize acid, since they contain
minerals that are acid binding.

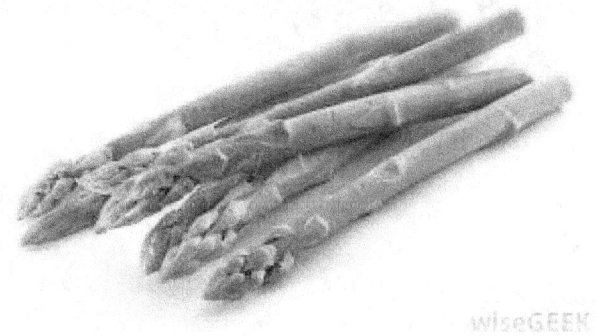

Vegetables at 93% Acid Binding – best vegetables to eat
Kelp, Seaweed, Watercress, Asparagus

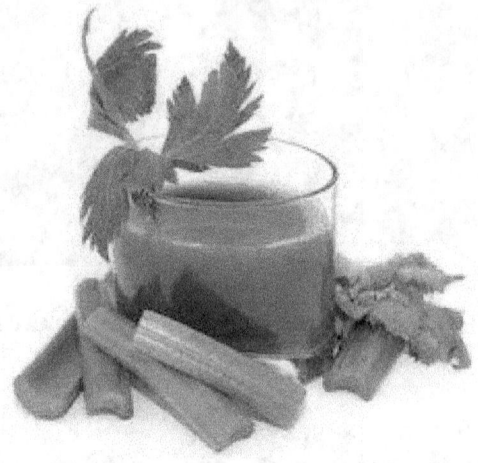

Vegetables at 80% Acid Binding – Still the best to eat
Lettuce Leaf, Oyster plant, Pumpkin, Spinach, Squash, Peas,
Carrots, Celery, Chard, Swiss, Dandelion greens

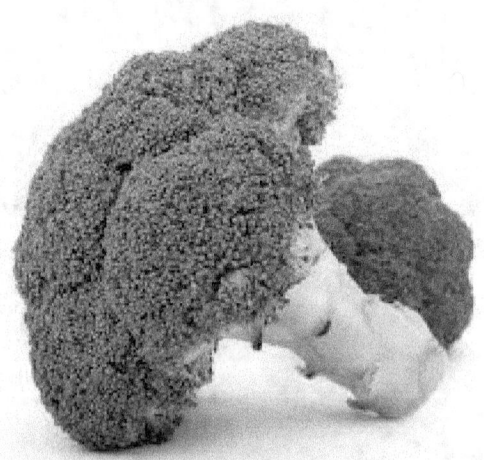

Vegetables at 73% Acid Binding – Great vegetables to eat
Bamboo shoots, Beets, Broccoli, Cabbage, Cauliflower,
Collards, Corn, sweet, Ginger (fresh), Mushrooms, Mustard
greens, Onions, Pepper, Potatoes, Green, Lima, String beans,
Potatoes

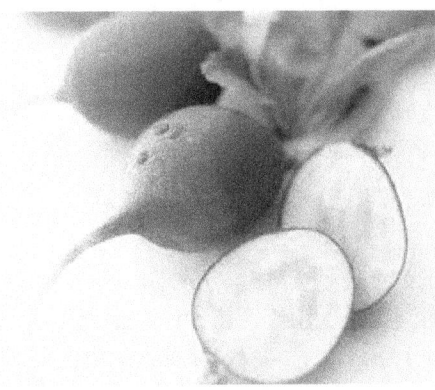

Vegetables at 67% Acid Binding – eat plenty of these Brussels sprouts, Cucumbers, Eggplant, Okra, Onions, Radishes, Tomatoes

Vegetable juices at 80% to 93% Acid Binding Parsley, wheat grass, carrot, celery, etc.

Soy Bean Products at 60% Acid Binding – limit your use of tofu since it is a genetically modified organism, GMO Dried beans, Soy cheese, Soy milk, Tempeh, Tofu

Other Foods For Gout

Here are some other misc. foods to eat that are acid binding. Starches at 80% Acid Binding

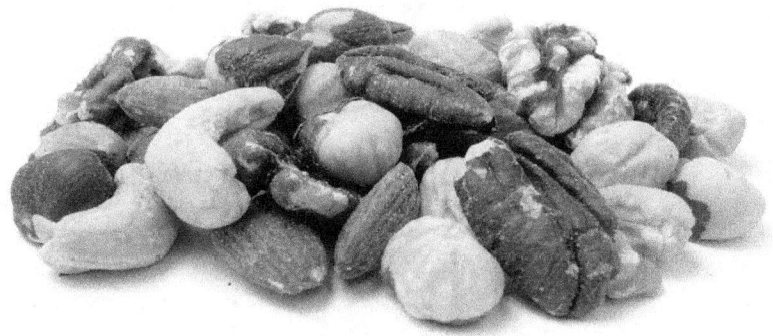

Nuts and Seeds at 60 % to 67% Acid Binding

Almonds, sesame seeds, Granola, Essene Bread, Chestnuts

Misc. foods at 60% Acid Binding

Horseradish, Amaranth, Millet, Quinoa, Dried beans, Soy cheese, Soy milk,

The following foods are alkaline binding, which means that they create acids that will bind with alkaline salts and remove them from your body. These foods when eaten in excess will create an acid body.

You should only eat around 20% of these foods in your diet, and the other 80% should come from fruits and vegetables or foods that are acid binding.

NOTE: The lower the alkaline binding percentage, the more that food is acid producing.

Oils

All oils are basically at 50% and are considered neutral. This includes almond, avocado, canola, coconut, corn castor, olive, soy, sunflower oil, etc.

Food That Creates Acid

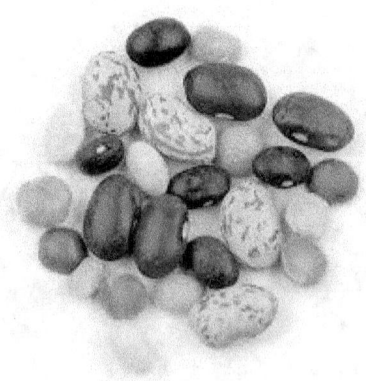

Beans, starches, and nuts and seeds at 40% to 46% Alkaline Binding and create body acid.

Aduki, Black, Broadbean, Garbanzo, Mung, Pinto, Barley, Corn Meal, Lentils, Brans, Cashews, Coconut (dried), Pecans, Brans, Millet, Filberts, Walnuts, Pumpkin, Sunflower
Starches at 26 to 33 % Alkaline Binding or highly acidic

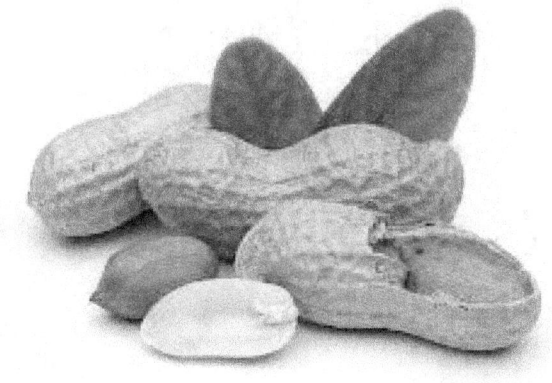

Brown Rice, Buckwheat, Oats, Spelt, Wheat Whole, Peanuts, corn, rye

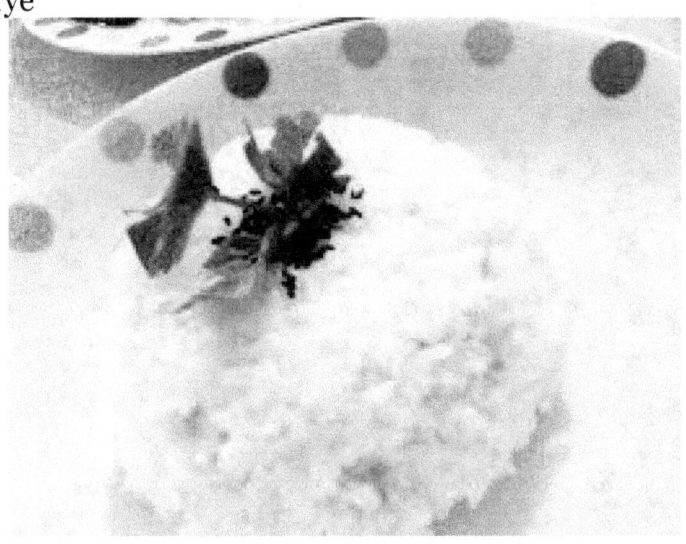

Rice at 20% Alkaline Binding and highly acidic, White rice

Sugar at 13% Alkaline Binding, highly acidic
White beet or cane sugar

Meat and Fish

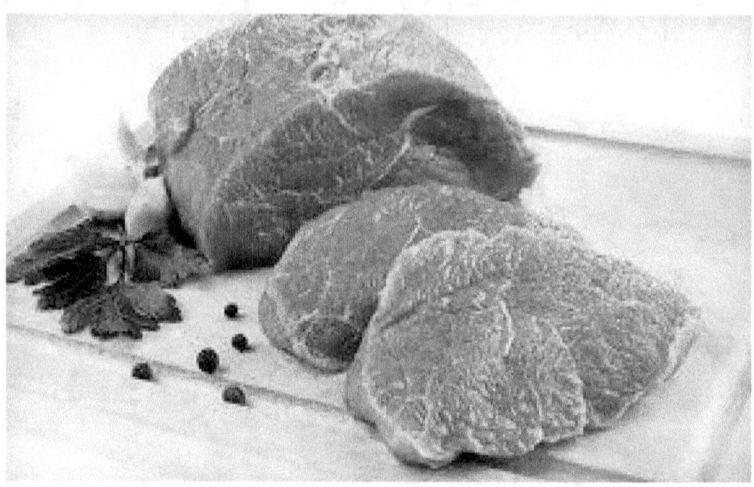

Meat at 26% alkaline binding highly acidic
Fish With fins and scales, Shellfish - shrimp, scallops, crab lobster, oyster
Meat at 20% Alkaline Binding, highly acidic

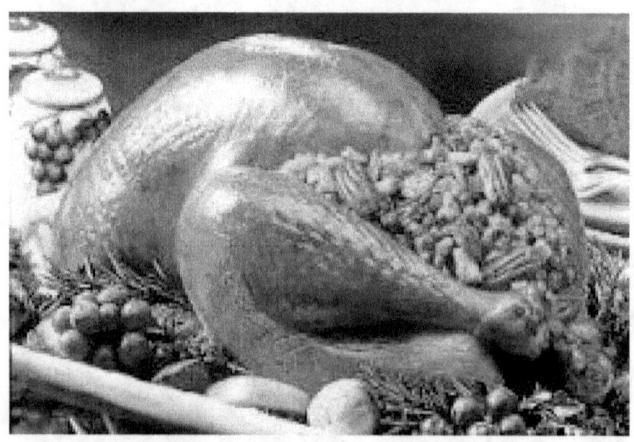

Chicken, turkey, rabbit
Meat at 13% Alkaline Binding, highly acidic

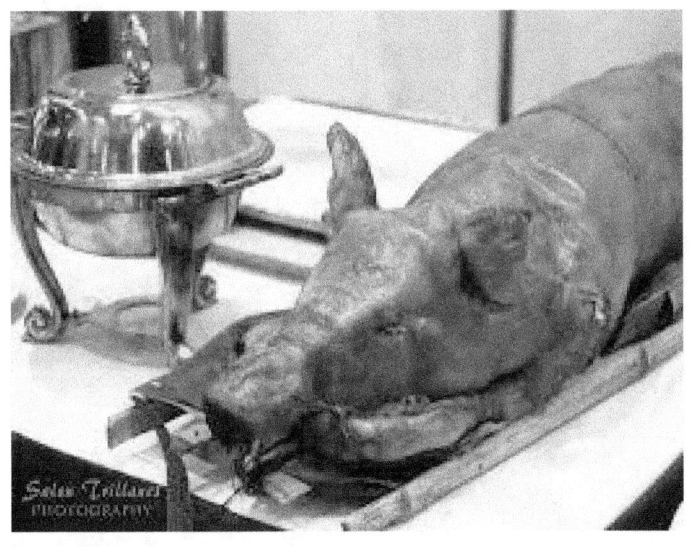

Beef, goat, pork, lamb

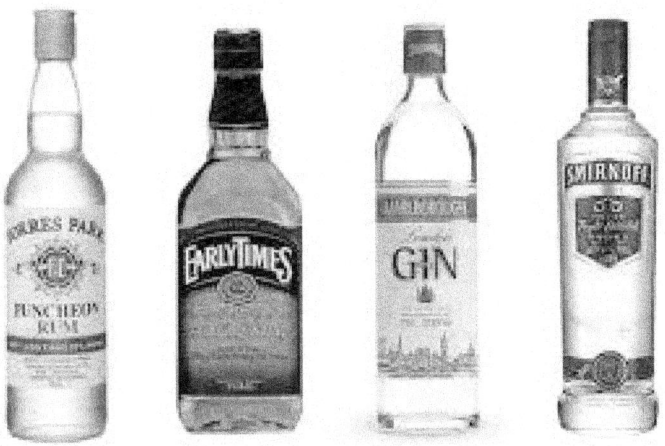

Misc. Products at 13% to 26% Alkaline Binding highly acidic Liquor, wine, beer, coffee, black tea, caffeine drinks

8: A Body Cycle Reduces Gout

Body cycles are time periods where your body is doing certain functions in your body. It does this automatically, as if it was on a timer. Knowing what these functions are, will help you get relief from your disease and even eliminate it.

Here are the 3 natural body cycles:

There are three natural body cycles, but the most important one for your gout is cycle 1.

Cycle 1 time period: 4 a.m. to noon

This cycle is the time where your body is eliminating toxins, acids, wastes, and derby through urine, bowel movements, and other secretions. Most people interfere with this cycle, since they are unaware of it, causing constipation, increase weight and various detrimental illnesses.

During the elimination cycle, 4 a.m. to noon, eat and drink only fruits and their juices or vegetable juices. For breakfast, eat a bowl of fruits or have a fruit smoothie made with apple juice, banana, and fruits in season.

Before noontime, eat fruits as snacks. Forty-five minutes before noon, eat your last fruit. You can eat and drink all the fruits and juices you want up to noontime.

Fruits contain the right balance of nutrients, with about 70% distilled water. Eat them without cooking them. They are easy to digest and absorb and do not stress your colon. They activate peristaltic action in your colon and help you have a bowel movement.

Use the Acid Binding fruits listed in the previous chapter. Here are some more fruits to eat:

Apples

Apricots

Avocados

Bananas

Blueberries

Boysenberries

Cantaloupes

Cherries

Figs and dates

Grapes

Grapes

Lemons

Nectarines

Oranges

Papayas

Peaches

Pears

Persimmons

Plums

Prunes

Raspberries

Strawberries

Watermelons

Eat all melons together and not with other fruit, and wait 1/2 hour before eating other fruit. Melons require specific enzymes to be digested in your stomach, so other fruits eaten with melons will just sit in your stomach, waiting to be digested. This will cause you gas and an acid stomach.

Eating Solid Food for Breakfast

Eating solid food for breakfast – eggs potatoes, rice, meat, cereal, milk, and so on, the typical breakfast, interferes with your body's elimination cycle and eventually leads to sickness and excess weight.

It takes over 3 hours to digest heavy and solid food. The food you should be eating in the morning should digest quickly. This helps you to activate peristaltic colon action to create a bowel movement and to continue your body's detoxification and elimination process.

Heavy food slows down the elimination of toxins from your body, and this causes fecal matter and toxins to remain in your colon longer than necessary. These toxins then get stored in your body, as fat and acids.

It takes 1 to 1 1/2 hour or so to digest fruits and fruit juices. Because of this, they help to cleanse your body of waste during the time from 4am to noontime.

So if you are not already having fruits and fruits and vegetables juices for breakfast and snacks, start slowing changing your eating habits. This will help you detoxify your body daily, lose weight, create an alkaline body, and eliminate your gout.

9: Use This Program to Stop Gout

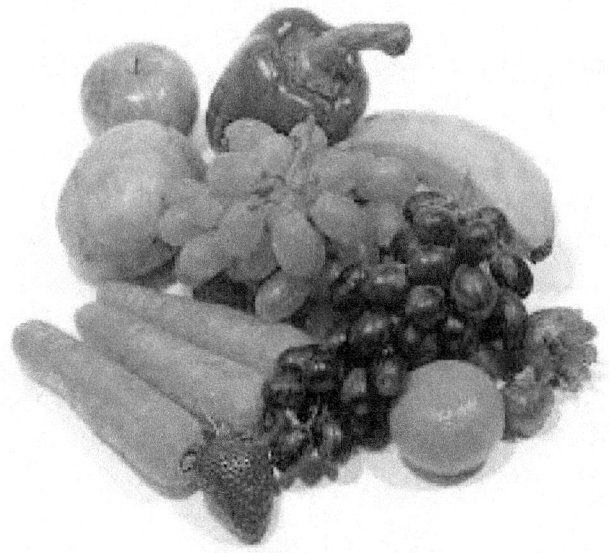

I provided you with a lot of information on various aspects of gout. This gives you a chance to see what action you need to take, to get rid of it and to cure it.

I have given many things to do and natural remedies and supplements to take. The reason for this is so that you can first find those remedies that you might already have in your kitchen or refrigerator. If you have these foods or remedies, you can get started right away, getting some pain relief.

One of the secrets of curing gout is using the idea that gout is an acid-alkaline imbalance. So, what this means is that you need to stop eating and doing those things that are causing this imbalance in your body.

What this imbalance means is that you have too much acid in your body, which causes uric acid to precipitate out of your blood and create crystals that end up in your joints.

Here is an outline of how to get started.

- Start drinking more water. You want to urinate more to reduce the amount of uric acid you have in your body.

- You want to drink fruit and vegetable juices that give you more acid binding minerals, like watermelon, various juices, fruits, and herbal remedy teas. Use more fruits and vegetables that give you 80 to 100% acid binding results.

- You need to get rid of the excess acid in your body. So you need to do the three-day colon **and blood cleanse.** This cleanse will pull out your excess body acids in your blood, lymph liquid, and around and inside your cells.

Make some changes in the way you eat.

- Look at the list of foods to avoid. You don't have to be perfect here, just start minimizing their use.

- Then look at the food to eat more of and start adding them into your diet.

Start using some of the natural remedies. Look over the list and choose a couple of them.

- Pick a couple of them and use them for a week to see if you see a difference in your condition. Keep trying different ones, until you find one that works for you. You can do short time test, to see if any of remedies give you quick relief.

Now take a look at the various supplements that are good for gout.

- Use kelp and celery seeds to help reduce body acid.

- Use digestive enzymes to help you digestion your food better, so that you don't create a lot of stomach acid waste.

Gets pH paper so you can see how acidic you are.

- Use pH paper for a few months, so you can monitor your condition and progress.

Creating a more alkaline body will go a long way in improving your overall health.

Read over the section on Burning Acid. There is a chart there that tells you the best fruits and vegetables to eat to create an acid body. You need to concentration on this produce.

For example, here are the top fruits to eat:

- Fruits at 100% Acid Binding – Best fruits To Eat Lemons, melons – any type, watermelon

- Fruits at 93% Acid Binding – great fruits To Eat Cantaloupes, dried dates, dried figs, limes, mango, papaya

But don't neglect the other fruits.

For the top vegetables to eat here is the start:

- Vegetables at 93% Acid Binding – best vegetables to eat Kelp, Seaweed, Watercress, Asparagus

Vegetables at 80% Acid Binding – Still the best to eat
Lettuce Leaf, Oyster plant, Pumpkin, Spinach, Squash, Peas,
Carrots, Celery, Chard, Swiss, Dandelion greens
There is still one more important thing to do:
- Change the way and what you eat for breakfast.

In the Body Cycle chapter, I go over how to eat breakfast.
- Use the best fruits or vegetables for breakfast.

This will help you to detoxify your body and eliminate and
neutralize acids daily. This one of the best health practices you
can do for your body.

There you have it, a comprehensive health program that is
super for getting rid of gout and giving you better overall
health.

Use these principles and you will gain new health and
happiness.

10: Other Resources

Get one of my best kindle books *free* below:

http://www.natural-remedies-thatwork.com

Kevin is a natural consultant nutritionist educated in the United States in Nutrition.

Resource page

Here are some of the other kindle e-books about natural remedies that are recommended by this author. You can see the entire list at:

http://tinyurl.com/b2f7wd3

Constipation Remedies

Best Constipated Women Natural Cures

Essential Fatty Acids
Taking The Mystery Out Of Essential Fatty acids
Amazing Fish Oil Benefits Revealed

Nutrition Remedies
Magnesium Nutrition Revealed
Potassium Health Secrets Revealed

Stomach Remedies
Acid Reflux: Fast and Easy Cures For Acid Reflux
How To Do Natural Colon Cleansing

Misc. Remedies
Iron Deficiency Anemia
What Is A Hiatus Hernia?
HerniaBest Varicose Vein Treatments?

Men's Health
Best Impotence Health Diet

Weight loss
Ten (10) Day Quick Success Weight Loss Program

To see all of the kindle books written by this author, go to the Authors Profile Page or this URL:

http://tinyurl.com/b2f7wd3

If you need support or want to promote any of his e-books, please contact him at rss41@yahoo.com and expect a reply within 24 hours.

Give A Review

And, don't forget to give a review for this e-book at Amazon. It's not hard to give a review. It can be only a sentence or two. You don't have to leave a long review. A short review helps other people decide if they want to buy a book. So give a short review and give your thoughts to help other people and to help the author improve his book.

Here's to your health,

Kevin Reed